The Lazy Person's Guide to Exercise

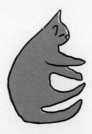

OH EDITIONS

DEDICATED TO EVERYONE WHO THINKS EXERCISE OR ANY FORM OF SELF-CARE IS NOT FOR THEM BECAUSE THEY'RE NOT WORTH IT – IT IS, AND YOU ARE!

The Lazy Person's

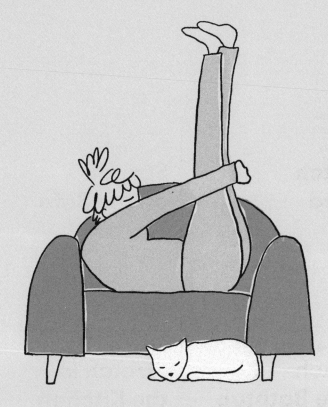

Guide to Exercise

Susan E. Clark

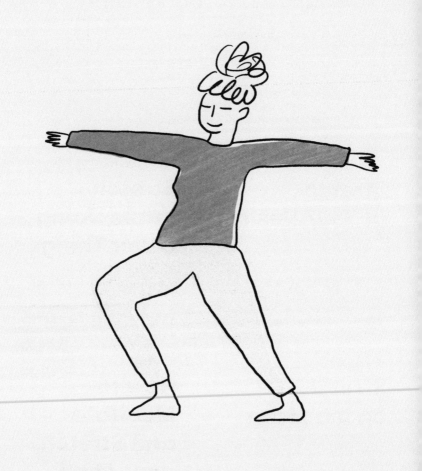

INTRODUCTION

Simple stretching is the new way to get your body toned – and the good news is that you don't even have to get out of bed or off your chair to do it.

According to research, stretching is important for keeping our muscles strong and our joints flexible.

And it turns out that stretching is just as important as aerobic fitness or building muscle, because muscles that are not stretched get shorter and tighter, which can lead to injury when we ask the body to do even the simplest of everyday tasks like reaching for the sprinkles at the back of the baking cupboard or lifting the shopping out of the car.

Exercise scientists stress it's important that we stretch and move our bodies every day, but happily they don't say where we need to be when we move.

So, with a few tips and tricks up our sleeves, we can safely move our bodies any time, any place, and don't even have to leave our homes to get the benefits of stretching.

If you're now starting to think, *Oh . . . I don't know. I'm pretty lazy, and this sounds like a step too far for me*, don't panic! You're not expected to stretch every single muscle, every day. But if you can find just 10 or 15 minutes a day to work your way through the simple and fun stretching exercises in this book, you'll quickly start to feel the benefits.

You'll walk and feel taller, and you'll know you can always rely on your body to do what you ask of it.

FLEXERCISE SCIENCE

Sadly, a sedentary lifestyle is not the only reason we lose the range of movement and flexibility that we are all born with.

Our bodies dehydrate and stiffen with age – so much so that by the time you are an adult, you've lost 15 per cent of the moisture content of your tissues, which makes you less supple and more prone to injury.

As a result, our muscles shrink and lose mass, and the muscles that were once elastic and springy get caught up with the thick connective tissues that connect them and, as a result, become less and less yielding and more and more inflexible.

Stretching helps slow this process by pulling apart these cellular "cross-links" that should not be there. It also stimulates the production of calcium, which acts as a tissue lubricant to prevent muscles from drying out and allows our muscles to rebuild the way they were always intended to be.

And, apart from all the physical benefits, a slow, focused stretching session can help relax you and reduce stress. Who knew something so simple could be so powerful? With all those benefits, you'd be mad not to do it.

Finally – as with any new form of exercise, it's best to talk to your doctor if you have any concerns.

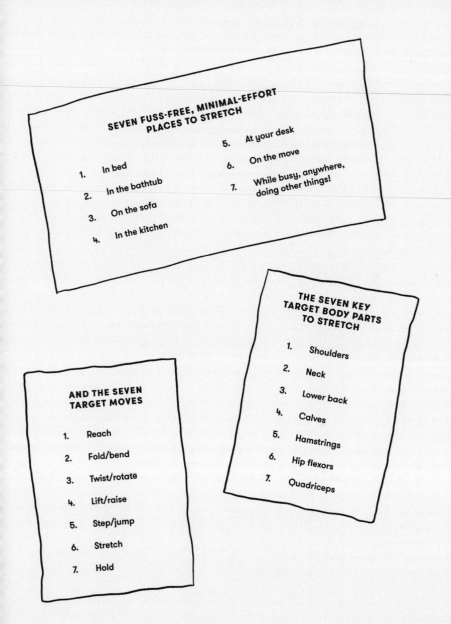

SEVEN FUSS-FREE, MINIMAL-EFFORT PLACES TO STRETCH

1. In bed
2. In the bathtub
3. On the sofa
4. In the kitchen
5. At your desk
6. On the move
7. While busy, anywhere, doing other things!

THE SEVEN KEY TARGET BODY PARTS TO STRETCH

1. Shoulders
2. Neck
3. Lower back
4. Calves
5. Hamstrings
6. Hip flexors
7. Quadriceps

AND THE SEVEN TARGET MOVES

1. Reach
2. Fold/bend
3. Twist/rotate
4. Lift/raise
5. Step/jump
6. Stretch
7. Hold

HOW TO USE THIS BOOK

This book is all about flexibility, and how much that improves depends on how, when and for how long you do these exercises.

With seven target muscle groups, seven different stretch moves and seven different places to stretch your way to fitness, there are a lot of different combinations, and a lot of ways to very easily integrate them into your life.

Here are some suggestions to get you started, but feel free to come up with your own schedule, because you know what your body likes best.

1. You can choose one target muscle group, one target location and one muscle move per day.

2. Or you can choose your location and then decide which of the seven stretch exercises (or, as I like to call them, *flexercises*) designed for that locale you want to do for your session, which allows you to specifically target the muscles you want to work on. For example, if you've spent a long day sitting down for work or travel, you may want to choose stretches that work on your hamstrings or on loosening a stiff lower back.

3. Or, you may prefer to stay in one location and, if time allows, work your way through all seven target areas to give yourself a top-to-toe stretchtastic workout.

4. You could also choose the types of movement you think your body will enjoy on a particular day. For example, if you plan to stretch first thing in the morning then stretch, reach and twist moves will be good to warm your joints and muscles for the day ahead.

Each stretch is designed to complement the ones before and after it, but they work equally well on their own. With these stretches you can do as much or as little as you like, although if you want to see some benefits soon then try to do 30 minutes of stretching at least three times a week. That said, you could do just 15 minutes every day for six days instead and take a rest day before you start your stretching regimen again in a new week.

And since we're all about keeping things simple and making life easy, you can even watch Netflix or multitask at your desk while you practise some of your stretching exercises.

Now you know the theory and the structure behind the stretches, let's dive right in to your first set of stretches.

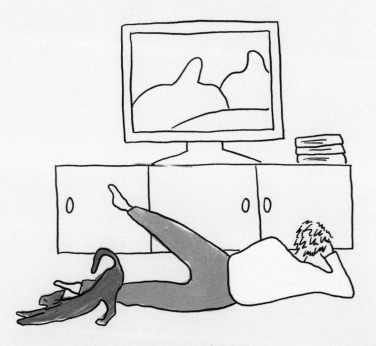

Stretch in Bed

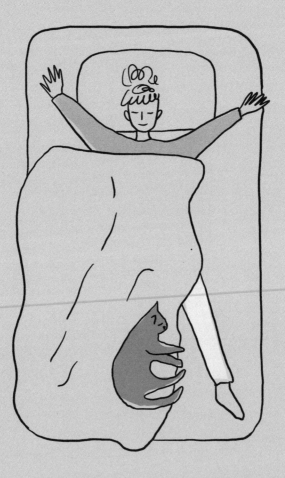

1.

Is there any better place to relax and give your body the gift of a feel-good exercise session than the comfort of your own bed?

It's the perfect way to start your day – you can stretch out in the morning sunshine, with a new day of possibilities ahead of you. And all you need is an extra 30 minutes under (or, when needed, on top of) the covers to give your body a gentle stretch workout.

It's worth noting that if you've not stretched your body for a while, always move gently and cautiously test your limits. We don't want any injuries!

#1   **Become a Pencil**

This is a delicious full body stretch – and as you
stretch into being the longest and leanest possible
version of you, the body's internal organs get
a healthy stretch out too.

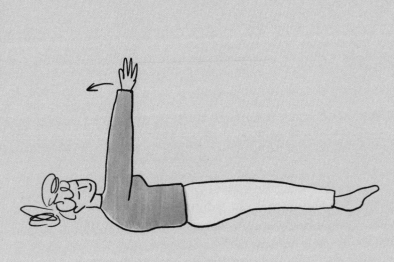

→ Lie on your back. As you
  inhale, raise both arms
  up alongside your head.

→ Keep the elbows tucked
  in alongside the ears, and
  once you are in position,
  stretch by reaching even
  further to make your body
  longer. Exhale.

→ Now imagine your ankles
  being gently pulled to
  stretch out your middle
  torso and your legs.

→ Breath in, and in your
  mind's eye see your whole
  body stretching out in
  one long line from head
  to toe.

WORKS ON ⤵

The shoulders
and lower spine.

COMFY TIP

A full body stretch can
put strain on your lower
back. If this is the case
for you, pop a pillow
or cushion under your
back for extra support.

If this is still a little
uncomfortable, raise
your knees and focus
solely on stretching
out your arms above
your head.

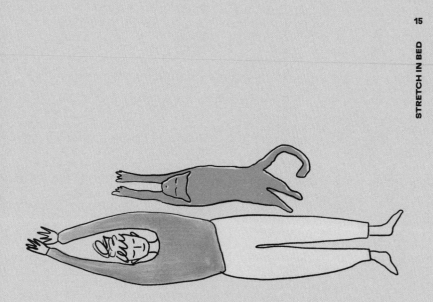

→ Stretch yourself out
as long as you can . . .
and then stretch just
a little bit more. Exhale.

→ At the edge of this
stretch, hold the breath
and count to 5 (then 10
and 20 as you progress).

→ Release the breath,
but remain lying
on your back for the
next bed exercise.

#2   Starfish and Swan

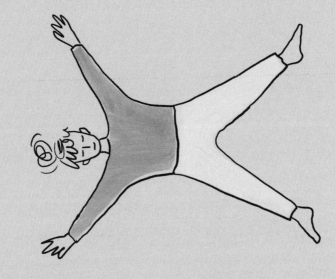

→ Start by lying on your back in a long line, like the Pencil stretch. Inhale and sweep both arms down to make a wide V shape. Stretch to your limit. Exhale.

→ Now, inhaling again, move both legs towards the bottom corners of your bed. Relax into the Starfish position.

→ Take a deep breath in and hold to a count of 5 (then 10 and 20 as you progress).

→ Exhale and relax. Take a moment to enjoy the sensation of your body waking up to the day, then bring your arms and legs back together in the Pencil stretch.

→ Repeat the Starfish bed stretch, but this time, when you have reached the edge of your stretch, close your eyes, inhale and slowly turn your head to the right.

WORKS ON ↴

Stretching and activating your
core abdominal muscles and
releasing built-up tension from
the neck muscles.

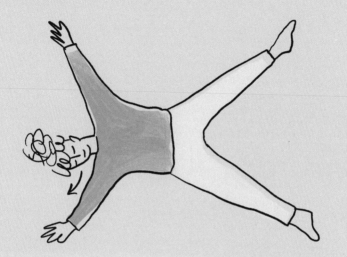

→ Really feel the stretch
in the top of your back.
You should also feel the
stretch down the opposite
side of your neck.

→ Breathe out and hold
the stretch for a count
of 5 (then 10 and 20
as you progress).

→ Inhale and turn your
head slowly back to
centre. Breath out as
you slowly turn your
neck to the left.

→ Repeat the neck turns
three times on each side.

→ At the end of the last
round, relax in the
Starfish stretch for
a count of 5 (then 10
and 20 as you progress).

→ Now bring your arms
to your sides and your
legs back together.

Lean on Me

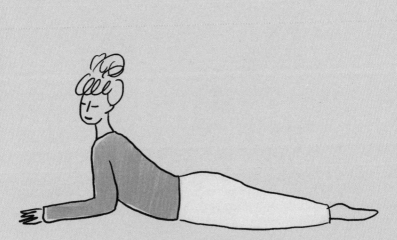

→ Flip over to lying on your stomach, turn your head to one side and take a few moments to feel the benefits of the first two bed stretches.

→ When you are ready, inhale deeply and raise the upper part of your body so you can rest, Sphinx-like, on your elbows, with your chin cradled in your hands. Exhale.

WORKS ON ⌐

Loosening the lower back.

THE BENEFITS OF A FLEXIBLE SPINE

— Stronger core
   muscles
— Less risk of back
   pain and injury

— Better posture
— Better balance
— A supple spine
   is a happy spine!

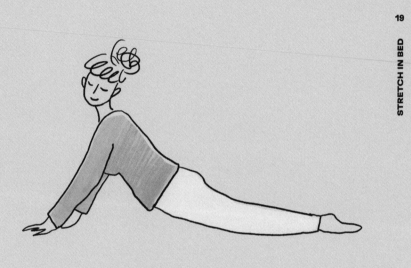

→ As you rest easy in this
  leaning posture, focus
  on how your lower back
  is stretching out and up
  to keep your upper body
  lifted and supported by
  your arms.

→ Imagine each of the
  vertebrae that make up
  your spinal column opening
  and stretching out to keep
  your spine supple.

→ Rest and breath in this
  position, holding to
  a count of 5 (then 10
  and 20 as you progress).

Folding Your Pyjamas (While Still Wearing Them!)

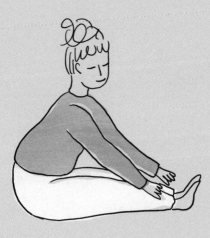

→ Sit up tall on your bed, making sure your legs are stretched straight out in front of you.

→ Take a couple of deep, calming breaths in this sitting position, then stretch your feet as far away from you as you can.

→ You will feel a stretch that starts to relieve any built-up tension (especially from walking) in both calves.

→ Take a moment to enjoy flexing your ankles up and down. When you're ready to start the stretch, close your eyes, take a deep breath in and, as you do so, raise your arms up above your head, keeping your elbows alongside your ears.

→ Hold to a count of 5, and as you exhale, slowly fold your body in half.

WORKS ON ↴

Stretching out the lower back, hamstrings and calves

FOLDING TIP

I can't help much with advice on folding laundry, but when it comes to folding your body, all you have to remember is to *let* it fold.

Always fold from the hips, never the waist.

Use your breath to work *with* your body to soften all the muscles in the lower back, which will then allow you to comfortably and effortlessly fold in half.

Easy!

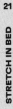

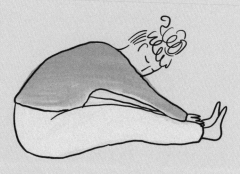

→ With your eyes still closed, see this as a fold that starts from the hips (not the waist). Do not force or strain to fold – just allow it to happen as your body relaxes.

→ If you can, reach forward to hold your toes with your fingers. If not, just gently take hold of your shins but not the ankles or knee joints.

→ As you rest a moment in your fold, focus on your breath and notice how with each exhale your body relaxes a little more deeply into the fold and your head drops closer to your knees.

→ Stay down in this folded position and enjoy feeling how deeply you are now breathing.

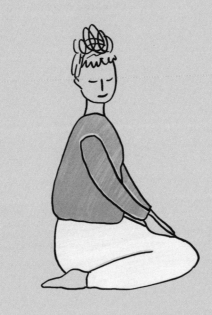

→ Stay on top of the bed
   covers but turn over so
   you are kneeling upright
   and facing the headboard
   (if you have one).

→ Take a deep breath in and
   slowly stretch forwards
   to bring your forehead
   down to rest on the bed.

→ Let each arm relax by the
   side of your body, close
   your eyes and wallow in
   the feeling you are back
   in your mother's womb,
   in a position you would
   have been familiar with
   back then.

→ Imagine you're in the
   womb, and all you can
   hear through the muffled
   sounds of the external
   world is the comforting
   heartbeat of your mother.

WORKS ON ⌐

Gently stretching out the hamstring muscles that run from the knee up the thighs at the back of the legs. But, just as importantly, this gorgeous stretch works instantly to calm the mind and nervous system – so you can use this move any time you feel anxious or stressed.

BETTER THAN ANY SPA TREATMENT!

If you have a partner or roomie you trust, you can invite them to deepen and extend this stretch by placing the base of one hand on the top of your spine and the base of their other hand in the middle of your lower back.

By applying a gentle pressure through both hands, they will lengthen your spine and deepen the stretch.

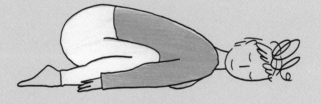

→ Allow your breath to come and go as it pleases Keep your eyes closed and sink into this deeply relaxing stretch, which should release the tension from the lower back and the top of the backs of the legs (both of which you stretched out in the previous fold).

→ Stay here as long as you like – unless you have a family or work deadline to meet!

→ It may not feel much like it, but you are doing excellent physical and psychological work here.

Why Stand When You Can Lie Down?

You know how you always see runners standing on one leg and bending the other at the knee to warm the muscles? Well, you're going to do the exact same thing, but – because we love things to be easy – you're going to do it lying face down on your bed. Genius!

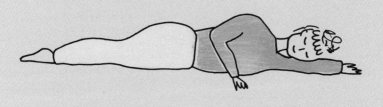

→ Lie face down on your bed and turn your head to the right-hand side so you can breathe.

→ Bend your right knee to raise the bottom half of your right leg up behind you and catch hold of your right ankle with your right hand.

→ Now breath and relax into a deep and delicious stretch of your quadriceps muscles.

WORKS ON ⅂

Lengthening the quadriceps (quads), which are the huge muscles that run up the front of the leg from the knee to the thigh.

WHY WE JUST LOVE OUR BEDS

While you sleep, your body is busy making an important hormone called melatonin, which controls the body's sleep/wake cycle. It also makes you feel comfy and relaxed. Levels of production drop off once daylight comes into the room (which is why it's important to sleep in the dark), but this is gradual, so your melatonin levels are still higher in the morning than they will be later in the day. That's why we all, quite naturally, want to curl up and cling to the cosy covers.

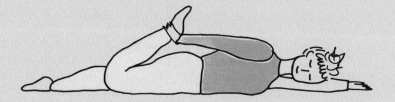

→ Allow your breath to slow and settle into a calming and natural rhythm and hold this stretch for a count of 5 (then 10 and 20 as you progress).

→ When you are done stretching out the right side, simply repeat on the left.

#7 The Leaping Frog...
Who Never Leaps

It's time to channel your inner Kermit! This move may feel a bit silly, but your body – especially your hips – will really thank you.

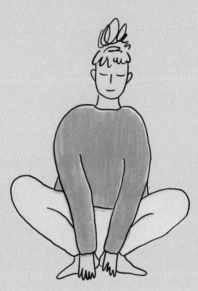

→ If you've been resting in the previous stretch, you need to bring yourself up to an upright kneeling position. With your hands stretched out in front of you for balance, squat on the tips of your toes with your heels together. This will open up the hips.

→ Put your fingertips onto the bed for extra balance – you should now resemble a ready-to-leap frog. Keep the heels together, close your eyes and open the groin area as widely as you can, pushing your knees out to the sides.

→ Tilt your head up so your throat stretches. Try to stay still for as long as you can.

Opening up the hips by stretching the hip extensor muscles, which will often feel very tight when you first begin to stretch them.

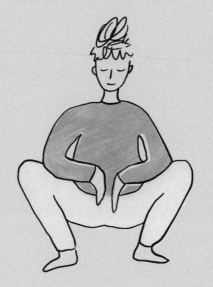

→ Experiment by pressing your elbows against the inner top part of each leg to further push the knees out.

→ Hold, and really take the time to enjoy this powerful move.

→ Sadly, it's now time to get up and start your day. The good news, however, is that your body is now nicely stretched, warmed up and more than ready for whatever the day throws at you!

Stretch in the Bathtub

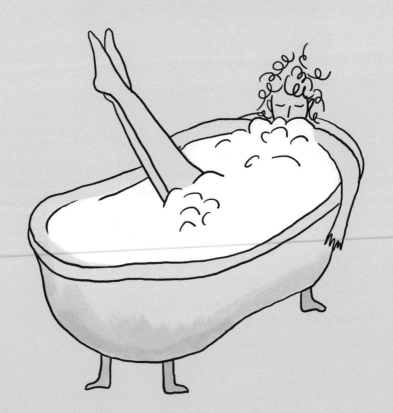

2.

We've all seen a cat, lying in a puddle of sunshine, stretching its whole body out ... and it just looks like the best, most luxuriously satisfying thing ever. Stretching and luxuriating go hand in hand, so the good news is you'll already be doing your muscles a favour by just sinking into a deep bath and closing your eyes to shut out the world and relax.

Warmth – including warm water – works to dilate the blood vessels, which improves circulation. This in turn brings more oxygen and nutrients to your muscles, helping to bring their elasticity back.

Plus, the buoyancy of the bath will make some movements feel easier to do than on dry land.

So, if you really think about it, there's probably no better place to embrace lazy exercise – and really hold those deep stretches – than in your own bathtub!

STRETCHING YOUR SPINDLES

You're going to hear about your "spindles"
in this chapter, so here's a quick quiz question:

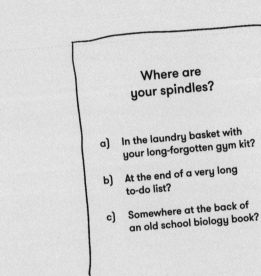

Where are
your spindles?

a) In the laundry basket with
   your long-forgotten gym kit?

b) At the end of a very long
   to-do list?

c) Somewhere at the back of
   an old school biology book?

The correct answer is . . . none of these.
Because while you may have studied biology at
school, I bet nobody told you about your spindles!

Our bodies have built-in "stretch detectors", known as muscle spindles, which most of us have never even heard of. They are very small sensory organs that run alongside our muscles and work to protect us from overstretching.

    With these exercises, we can deliberately target our stretch detectors and get them on board to allow for a greater (but still safe) stretch – and thus greater flexibility – while still protecting the muscles.

    But we can only do that once we know how. Which, handily, is what this section is all about . . .

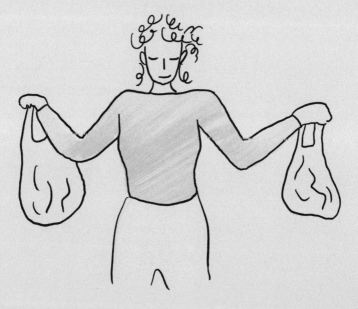

#1   **Rotating Chicken Wings**

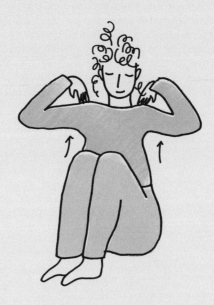

→ Sit upright on your
sitting bones and face
one end of the bath.
(If you're not sure where
your sitting bones are,
go and explore! Firmly
feel your bum cheeks with
your fingers and try to
find them - you're looking
for one on each side!)

→ Put your hands on your
shoulders, with the thumbs
at the back and the fingers
over the top, so your
elbows flare out. Pull your
elbows further up and back
so that you can really
feel the stretch.

→ Imagine these are your
little wings. We channeled
our inner frog before -
now it's time to channel
your inner chicken.

WORKS ON ⌐

The shoulder joints and the huge, diamond-shaped trapezius muscles in the upper back.

ENGAGEMENT TIP

Clucking might help you get into the "chicken spirit" of this stretch, but maybe shut the bathroom door and turn some music up so nobody else can hear you. They might think you're really gone clucking mad!

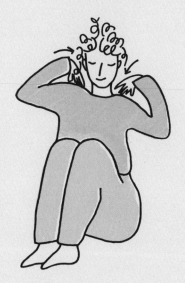

→ Inhale and rotate both "wings" backwards, allowing your chest to push out as you move your shoulders backwards, exhaling as you bring the arms forwards again.

→ The best way to really stretch into this movement is to close your eyes and envisage each of your elbows making wide circles in the air (in order for them to do this, you have to rotate the crucial shoulder cuff).

→ Once you get the hang of this movement, try to make those elbow circles as big as you can.

→ Rotate 5 times in one direction and then 5 times the opposite way (then 10 and 20 as you progress).

→ Really feel the shoulders and the muscles at the top of the back working and loosening to allow you to make these big movements.

Exploring the Deep

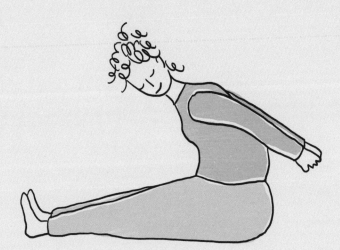

→ Once you have finished these shoulder rotations, put your arms behind your back and clasp your hands together.

→ Now fold yourself forwards and raise your arms into a stretch up and out of the shoulder joint.

→ This is not an easy movement, so don't force it – it might take some time to master this one. Just allow the arms to lift and the shoulder joint to open out.

→ Once you have reached the edge of your stretch, lift those arms a tiny bit more and then hold.

WORKS ON ⤵

All the muscles that support
the mid and upper back,
plus the shoulder joints.

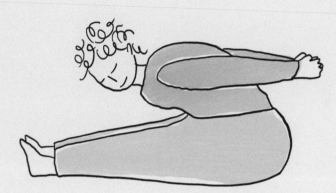

→ As you stretch down into
this position with your
arms up, imagine those
muscle spindles trusting
you enough to allow a
little more stretching.
Hold the stretch and
count to 5 (then 10 and
20 as you progress).

→ When you are done, bring
your arms down, lift your
folded body back up to
a sitting position and
slide back down into the
warm bath to reward all
the muscles that have
just worked so hard
for you.

Swan Stretch

This lazy flexercise will give all the muscles in your neck a longed-for release. And if you're streaming some funky bath-time music, you can sing along while you do this, making it your own, stretch-centric version of a swan song!

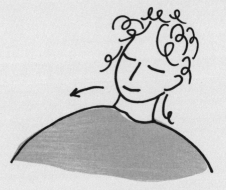

→ Stay supine in the bath, with your legs stretched out and your arms relaxed along your sides.

→ Close your eyes and bring your focus to your neck and throat areas.

→ Keeping your eyes closed, slowly turn your neck to the right. If your face goes into the water, don't worry – your eyes are closed and you won't be staying submerged for long.

→ Now bring your neck slowly back to the centre and start turning it to the left-hand side.

WORKS ON ⏆

The neck and upper back muscles, and also helps improve mood and mental health.

HEAVY IS THE HEAD

Did you know that an adult's head weighs around 5–6kg (11–12lb)? That's around 40 bananas, or 35 baseballs, or an Italian greyhound. And all that weight is resting on just seven vertebrae in your neck and supported by around 20 muscles.

No wonder, then, that the muscles of the neck and shoulders get so tense! Stretching them can prevent tension headaches, stiffness and general feelings of lethargy, so if you don't do any other stretches in (or out of) the bath, do these!

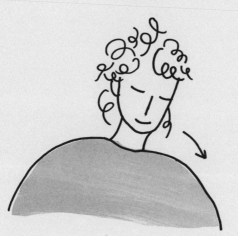

→ Again, keep your eyes closed, stretch as far as you feel comfortable and really feel the rotation of your neck and the support the water buoyancy is offering for that heavy head you've been carrying around all day.

→ Let go of your cares, letting the warm water melt them away each time you complete a full rotation of right-centre-left-centre.

→ If you're starting out, do just 5 full rotations, and build to 10 and 20 as you progress.

#4 Row, Row Your Boat (Singing Optional)

Your body should now be feeling ready for something a bit livelier, so you're now going to pretend you're rowing towards some distant shore – let's say it's the Greek coast. You're rowing to shore for a fresh lunch and chilled bottle of wine. Perfection.

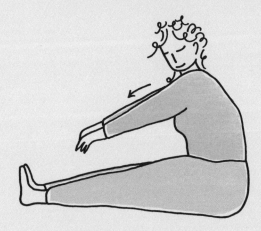

→ Find your sitting bones again (see Rotating Chicken Wings on page 32) and sit tall, making sure your spine is straight.

→ Imagine a piece of string attached to the top of your spine, which is gently being pulled higher. You should find yourself sitting taller, making sure you really lift those supporting muscles in the middle of the back.

→ Now close your eyes and imagine yourself in that little boat. Clench both hands with palms facing down out in front of you. Keep your elbows bent and tucked into your side (as if you are holding onto the oars).

→ Exhale as you bend forwards from the hips, straightening your arms as you do so.

WORKS ON ⤷

The muscles of the lower back.

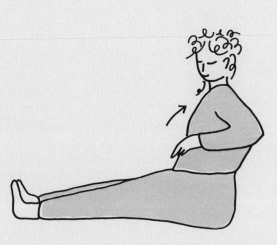

→ Inhale at the edge of the stretch then lean back as far as you can, drawing your clenched hands back towards your shoulders.

→ Keep your legs stretched out straight in front of you as you complete 5 rounds (then 10 and 20 as you progress).

→ Now reverse it! Imagine you need to backtrack to avoid a congregation of jellyfish. Complete 5 rounds (then 10 and 20 as you progress).

→ When you have finished, slide down into the warm water and rest.

#5 Cradle Stretching

This is the name I give to any stretch in which you are gently cradling a part of the body. Like if you were handling a small baby or a puppy, you need to be quietly coaxing and gentle. That's how you need to be for this cradling stretch – the main thing this flexercise calls for is for you to show these body parts some love.

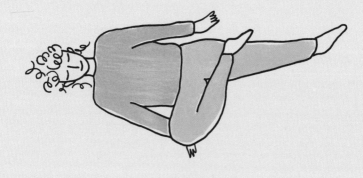

→ Find a comfortable position, then cross your right leg over your left so your ankle rests on your left thigh.

→ Make sure that you cradle the body parts you are moving to reassure them they are safe in your hands. Take hold of your right ankle and the side of your right foot and gently guide them into this position.

→ You are now going to use your left hand to flex the right foot, which will stretch the right calf muscles.

WORKS ON ⤵

The ankle joints and
the calves.

BEST FEET FORWARD

Try to remember your
poor feet. They give
you the stability and
foundation for all your
movements, and yet
too often people never
stop to even think about
stretching them.

Make this stretch
a regular part of your
practice and your feet
and ankles will reward
you by staying strong
and keeping you on
the move!

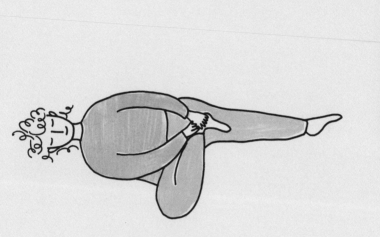

→ Cradle your right ankle
  with your right hand,
  and use your left hand
  to press the front of your
  right foot down. You will
  need to experiment a bit
  to get the pressure right,
  but remember to always
  proceed with caution
  and care.

→ Flex the right foot up
  and down 10 times, then
  switch legs and repeat.

→ Notice how this releases
  tension from the calves,
  allowing them to stretch
  out and relax. Remember to
  make each of your movements
  careful and cradling.

#6　The Funky Pigeon

Quick safety note: it's a good idea to use
a non-slip bath mat to stop you sliding
around during this exercise.

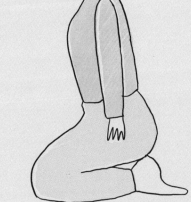

→ Adopt a kneeling position,
with your buttocks resting
on your heels and your
hands holding the sides of
the bath to keep you safe.

→ Make sure you are facing
one end of the bath, and
as you exhale, stretch
your left leg back out
behind you, keeping it
parallel to, and in line
with, your body. Your
right knee should stay
facing forwards.

→ Keeping your hands
shoulder-width apart,
move your arms forward
so your hands rest on
the bottom of the bathtub,
slightly in front of your
right knee.

→ Take a moment to settle
before moving into the
Funky Pigeon. To do so,
slide your left heel
a few inches to the right.
It should end up resting
on the right-hand side.

WORKS ON ⌐

Your hamstrings and quadriceps, so you can thank this clever pigeon for giving you two kick-ass muscle group benefits for the price of just one bathtub exercise!

EMBRACE YOUR INNER PIGEON

In some cultures, pigeons are seen as nothing more than flying rats, but in others pigeons are symbols of good fortune and prosperity. They're certainly a good thing as far as this stretch is concerned – it ranks in the top 5 stretches for those who spend their day sitting. It may even become one of your favourite lazy exercises, because it gives such a deep stretch to muscle groups that have probably been tense all day and are crying out for some R&R. So go on, embrace your inner pigeon.

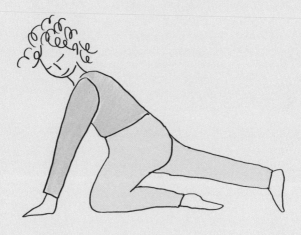

→ This gives your hamstrings and quadriceps an almighty stretch, and doing it in a warm bath means you should be able to stretch a little further than normal.

→ Keep your head up, facing forwards, and relax.

→ Hold for a count of 5 (then 10 and 20 as you progress).

→ Now bring yourself back to the original kneeling position and repeat on the other side, keeping the left leg bent and stretching out the right leg behind you.

SIDE SPLITS

The muscles that work to bring the hips together and stabilise our gait are called the hip adductors. These muscles support good balance and give us power, speed and alignment, as well as working to keep our hips flexible.

Hip flexors are those muscles near the top of the thighs that allow us to walk, kick, bend and swivel our hips, but these muscles – just like the adductors – can become too tight because we sit too long, have poor posture and don't take the trouble to stretch them.

You might never guess this, but tight hip adductors and flexor muscles can cause seemingly unrelated biomechanical issues that can really impact the quality of your waking life.

These include:
Lower back pain
Knee pain
Foot pain

Happily, the solution is to keep those muscles supple and healthy, and that can be achieved by exactly what we're doing here: stretching!

Hip flexors get stronger when they are bent or creased (which makes them contract), so that means squats and lunges if you're on *terra firma*. You'll be hard pressed to find anyone who actually likes a lunge (or a squat), so here are your bath time alternatives.

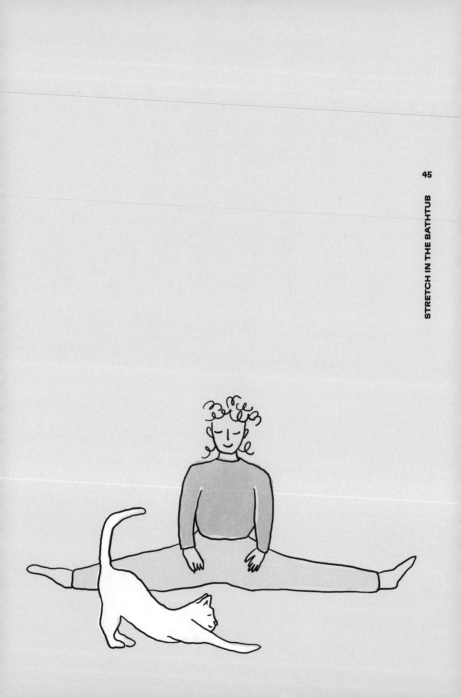

#7   Flexor Stretch

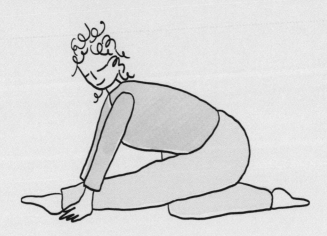

→ Half kneel with your
right foot on the bottom
of the bathtub. Your
right leg should be bent
at the knee and your left
leg should be stretched
out in front of you.

→ Balance and support your
body weight by resting
your hands on the bottom
of the bath.

→ Now lean forwards into
the stretch and really
feel the pull around the
groin and hip area.

→ Hold this stretch for
a count of 5 (then 10
and 20 as you progress).

→ Switch legs and repeat.

#8   Adductor Stretch

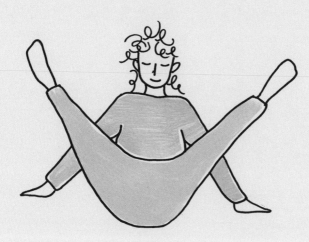

→ If you have a freestanding bath, you can dangle a leg over each side. If not, you'll need to sit sideways and dangle your legs over the edge.

→ Once you have both legs over the side(s), focus on stretching them as wide as you can. Settle into this stretch and really enjoy the sensation.

→ Push your legs as far apart as feels comfortable (don't be shy) and hold this stretch for a count of 5 (then 10 and 20 or more, as you progress) then bring your legs back into the bath.

→ Slide down into the warm soapy water and give yourself a gold star for doing the whole bathtub routine.

Stretch on the Sofa

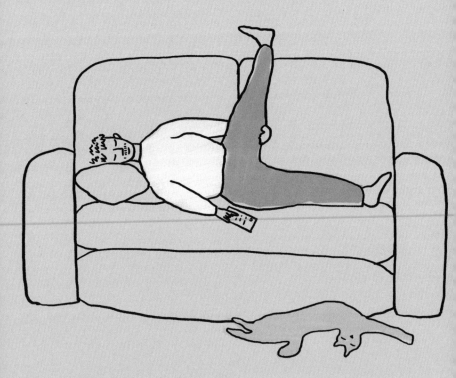

3.

According to recent research, Brits spend a whopping 44 days a year sitting on the sofa. Mind you, that research was carried out – obviously – by a furniture company. And they're probably not complaining about how much we all just love to sit down.

Americans, it seems, are not much better, spending an estimated 33 days with bums firmly glued to "couch" seats.

What are we doing when we're spending all this leisure time sitting? Probably not stretching. Probably binge-watching TV and scrolling on our phones.

But if ever there was an ideal place for us to multitask and move our bodies while doing all those other important things, then the sofa must be it. It's comfy, often squidgy, familiar, supportive and, for some of us, has become our best friend. As sad as that is.

So, let's introduce that best friend (the sofa) to the unexpected joys of flexercises, some of which require you to stay in your favourite position – lying down!

#1   The Big Bear Hug

It's a funny move, but stick with me, as you probably won't be laughing when you realise how effective this deceptively simple shoulder stretch is. With this stretch, the benefits are not in the movement itself but in the long deep hold I'm asking you to reach for.

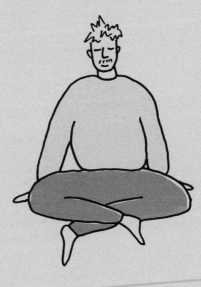

→ Find your sitting bones and sit nicely on the edge of your chosen sofa.

→ Imagine a hook coming down to catch a ring in the centre of your skull - like one of those hook-a-duck games at a fairground. Now imagine this imaginary hook pulling your upper torso up and into a straight line before we start. No spinal slouching allowed, or you won't get all the stretching benefits!

→ Now imagine you're on the platform at a railway station waiting to see someone you really love. What kind of hug would you give them?

WORKS ON ⌐

Shoulders and the muscles at the top of the back.

SHAKE, BABY

If this stretch is new for you, you may find your arms shaking if you stay in the hold position beyond a minute or so. This just tells you that your muscles, which are not used to working in this way, are tired and complaining.

Take this as a good sign! It means the stretch is doing the job: you are giving unused muscles a long overdue workout and stretch. But take care not to overdo it and cause injury. If you start to shake, focus on the breath, count to 5 if you can, then bring the arms back down.

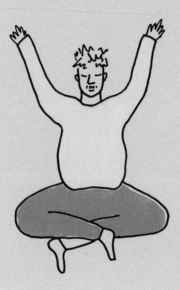

An enormous one! And that's what this stretch looks like: like someone is about to get a big bear hug from you.

→ With your spine straight, inhale and lift both arms up and out to the side to make a big V shape, with your neck and head at the centre.

→ Exhale and concentrate on raising your arms up as far as you can go.

→ Close your eyes and slowly count to 5 (then 10 and 20 as you progress).

→ Bring both arms back down and rest.

Rock and (Neck) Roll

Remember the side-to-side neck stretches you practised in the bath (page 36)? Well, these ingenious neck rolls complete the circle by stretching the neck forwards, sideways and backwards in a tension-releasing circular movement.

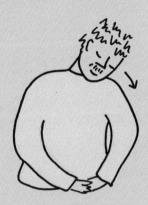

→ Stay sitting upright on the edge of the sofa, and try to keep your spine straight.

→ Drop your chin to the hollow at the bottom of the neck, rest for a few seconds, then slowly start to move your neck towards your right shoulder, keeping your chin in contact with your body as it moves.

→ Keep your breathing slow and steady and don't make any sudden jolts or jerks – imagine you're trying not to startle a skittish deer – but keep your neck moving slowly and purposefully.

→ Your neck should feel cradled by your shoulders and upper-back muscles.

→ When you reach your right shoulder, you will feel a deep stretch on the left side of your neck.

The neck and the muscles
that support the head.

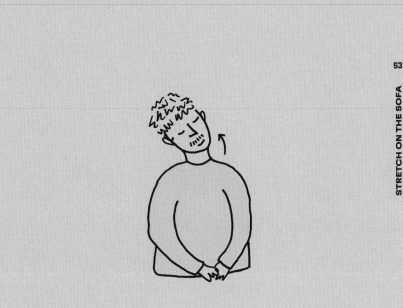

→ Don't drop your head
back too far or overextend
the neck but gently
sweep it around the
back towards the left
shoulder; it should
always feel supported.

→ At your left shoulder,
drop your chin back
down to your body, with
your chin back on the
centre line. This is
one complete neck roll.

→ If you have never done
this before, go slowly
and do just one round
to the right and then
a second round to the
left before stopping.
Build up to 5 rounds in
each direction (then 10
and 20 as you progress).

I Think I Knee'd a Hug

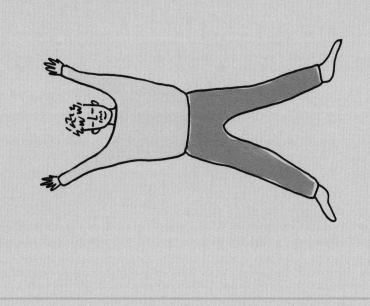

→ Lie down on your sofa and let your breath settle into a long, slow, deep rhythm. Maybe try not to actually fall asleep, but don't worry too much if you do – they say sleep is a healer!

→ If you've managed to stay awake, then you're going to give the lower back a delicious stretch just by raising both knees up and pulling them into your chest. If this blocks your view of the TV, then move the sofa!

WORKS ON ↴

Stretching out the lower back muscles.

ADDED VALUE

This stretch also gives your digestive tract a good massage so is great if you've had a heavy meal.

And if your lower back aches because you've been at your desk too long, you can also do this on the floor.

Lying on your back, keep your hands on your knees and make circles with the knees, first in one direction then the other. This will give the lower back a therapeutic massage, all while you elegantly resemble a flipped turtle.

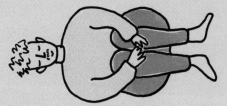

→ This folding of the body into itself will feel strange if you're a stretching newbie, but don't panic, the body and the breath will soon settle into this stretch so you can then hold it.

→ Hold for a count of 5 (then 10 and 20 as you progress).

→ When you have finished, unfold, let the legs stretch out on the sofa, and rest.

4

Toes Up

This exercise is so simple it's bound to become a firm favourite, and not least because the first instruction is . . . lie down. You'll nail it.

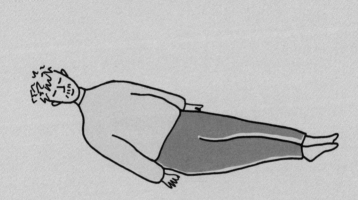

→ Once you're lying down, stretch your legs out in front of you on the sofa.

→ Turn on the TV. Told you you'd like this one.

→ Now, tilt both feet up and back towards the body at the exact same time. And hold. Feel that?

→ You should feel a deep stretch to the calf muscles in both legs, and it really is as simple as that.

WORKS ON ⤵

The calves and ankle joints.

READY TO SHOW OFF?

You can now stop calling the backs of your lower legs your "calves" and start referring to them as your "gastrocnemius" muscles. Everyone will be super impressed, and you'll instantly be invited onto everyone's pub quiz team. Probably.

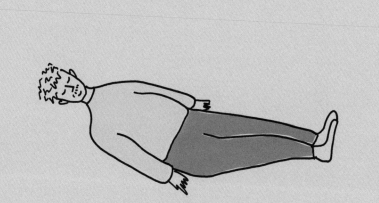

→ Breathe normally, carry on doing what you normally do on the sofa, but at the same time flex the ankles and tilt the feet back towards you 5 times (then 10 and 20 as you progress).

→ When you're done, you can rest.

#5   Prima Ballerina

This stretch may not sound like the most exciting, but it'll work wonders for strengthening the lower back and for releasing tension from the groin and the hamstrings. And while they may look super-simple, don't be fooled, because as you build to 10 and then 20 lifts, you'll start to really feel the power (and the burn) of a simple leg lift.

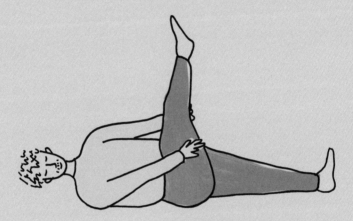

→ To start, lie back on the sofa and stretch both legs out in front of you.

→ Take hold of your right leg by putting both your hands on the muscles at the back of the leg, just below the knee, then use your hands and arms to lift the leg to a 90-degree angle.

→ Inhale and lift your leg, keeping your foot pointed like a prima ballerina.

→ Exhale, and as you hold this leg lift count to 5 (then 10 and 20 as you progress).

→ Now, keep your right hand on the back of your leg but move your left hand

WORKS ON ↴

The hamstrings and the core/abdominal muscles.

GOING DEEPER . . .

Once you've mastered this flexercise you can increase the intensity of the stretch by using a tea towel (or elastic exercise band, if you can find one gathering dust in the drawer) to flex the foot itself, which then works to stretch the calf muscles too.

Wrap the tea towel or band around the ball of the foot and gently pull the sides towards the upper body, which will work to bring the foot to a 90-degree angle and deepen the entire stretch. Just be wary of the elastic band snapping back in your face.

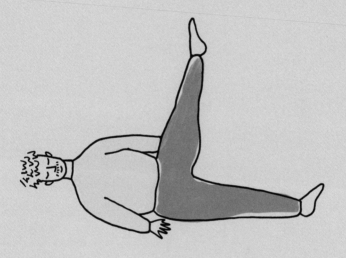

up to the middle of the hamstrings (at the top of that same leg) and gently pull the whole lifted leg closer to your chest. This works to really intensify the stretch.

→ Hold again for a count of 5 (then 10 and 20 as you progress).

→ Now swap legs so you are raising your left leg and stretching the hamstrings on that side of the body.

→ Repeat the same stretching sequence for your left leg, and when you've finished, rest with both legs stretched out on the sofa and a nice cup of coffee (or glass of wine) to hand.

#6 Scissor-Kick Lifts

The scissor-kick exercise works your core muscles, glutes, quads and adductors, so if you only have time for one sofa exercise, do this one.

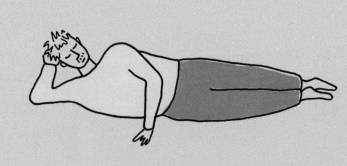

→ Lie on your left side, stretching out on the sofa to your full length.

→ Lift your head and rest it in your left hand, propped up by your left elbow.

→ Make sure you stay stretched out lengthways and make yourself as long as you can. Raise the right leg as high as you can without putting yourself out of alignment.

→ Do 5 scissor kicks of the right leg and then switch legs and sides.

WORKS ON ⤵

Tight hip flexors and
adductors (see page 44),
plus your core muscles,
glutes and quads.

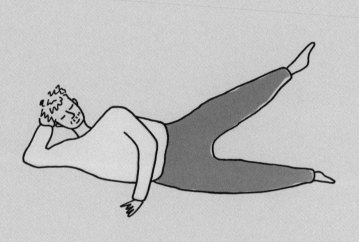

→ Once you switch, you'll
be facing the side of
the sofa (and probably)
away from the TV), so
don't be surprised if you
automatically and quickly
pick up the scissor kick
pace to get to the end of
your 5 lifts (then 10 and
20 as you progress).

→ When you start to think
you can't go on or do one
more scissor kick, take
a deep breath and prove
to yourself that you can.

→ When you've exercised
both legs this way,
you can go back to lying
on your back.

Lying Down Knee Bends

Your quadriceps can become too tight due to both over- and underuse. Sadly, the biggest culprits for underuse are work and sitting. Either way, let's fix the problem.

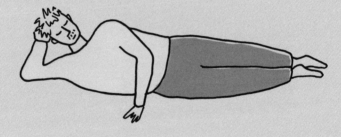

→ Lie on your left side, stretching out on the sofa to your full length.

→ Lift your head and rest it in your left hand, propped up by your left elbow.

→ Make sure you stay as stretched out as possible, and when you are ready, grasp the ankle of your right leg and fold that leg in half at the knee by bringing your heel in towards your buttock.

WORKS ON ⌐

The huge quadriceps muscles that run down the front of both legs.

SERIOUS HEALTH WARNING

Please don't skip this last sofa stretch. Weakened quads – or ones that are overworked and too tight – can cause serious lower back pain.

This is because they drag the entire pelvis down and throw the body out of its natural alignment. Tight quads can also cause knee pain. I'm sure you're starting to get the picture: ignore these at your peril. Thank you for coming to my TED Talk.

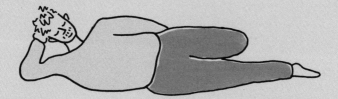

→ This is a powerful move, and if your quads are tight or weak you're not going to be able to hold for much longer than a count of 5 (then 10 and 20 as you progress).

→ Breathe normally as you stretch and hold then, when you are ready, switch sides to repeat with the left leg.

Stretch in the Kitchen

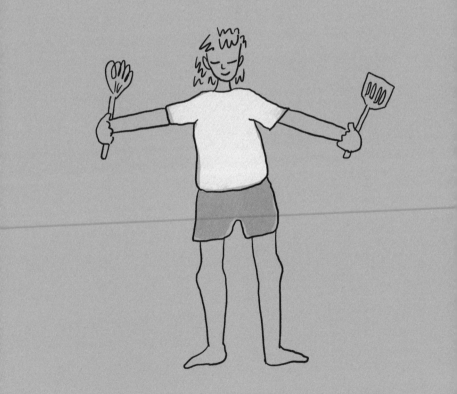

4.

Families – and even those living solo – still see the kitchen as the beating heart of their homes. And, since it's also a place where there's often lots of hanging around (waiting for the kettle to boil or the microwave to ping), it's also a great place to multitask and do some flexercises.

The average adult now spends just 60 minutes a day in the kitchen preparing their three daily meals. Researchers say this is half the time our parents typically spent slaving over a hot stove (lucky us), but it's still plenty long enough to get some quality stretches ticked off the "to-do" list. Less *Kitchen Nightmare* and more *Kitchen Dream*, I'd say.

#1   The Head Grab

This is a great flexercise to do while waiting for the kettle to boil, the custard to cool or the ready meal to ping.

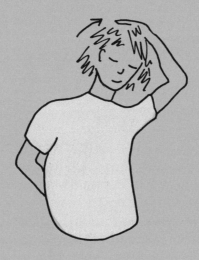

PART 1

→ Sit upright on a chair, on your "sitting bones" with both feet on the floor and your spine straight.

→ Rest your hands on your legs and close your eyes Take a slow, deep breath in, and as you exhale, slowly tilt your head down towards your left-hand shoulder.

→ Inhale slowly again and invite the neck to drop even further towards the shoulder, working with your body, not against it. I'm all about that positive collaboration.

→ Hold for 5, then repeat on the other side.

WORKS ON ↴

The muscles that support
the neck and head.

INVITATION TO STRETCH

Think of all these stretches
as an invitation to your
muscles rather than an
order. Remember, don't
ever strain to get into
a position.

After all, forcing the
body can cause injury,
and if you hurt yourself,
you won't want to stretch
again.

Allowing the body to
do what it would do
naturally – we can all
see how much a pet
cat or dog loves a good
stretch – means you
won't hurt yourself but
will soon start to enjoy
the sensation of giving
the body a good stretch.

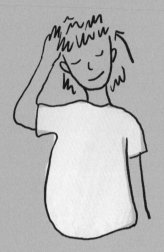

PART 2

→ You're now going to
repeat this gentle neck
stretch, but this time
you'll use your hands
to deepen the stretch.

→ So, before you tilt your
head to the left, place
your left hand on the
top, right-hand side
of the head.

→ Gently pull your head
down further towards
the shoulder.

→ Notice how even the
slightest pressure
from your hand deepens
the stretch.

→ Repeat on the other side.

#2　**Reach and Reward**

I don't want to boast, but I've invented a powerful psychological system. I know – impressive. It's called "Reach and Reward". A good reach deserves a good reward. Simple, but effective. Cue applause.

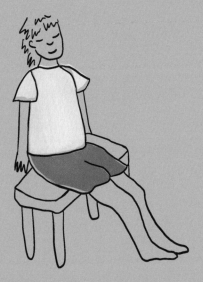

→ Preparation is key here. Firstly, choose a really good reward. Don't settle for a horrid "power" bar you bought in the health store – this needs to be a true treat or you just won't bother. I know what you're like.

→ Secondly, choose a clean countertop on which to place your chosen treat.

→ Finally, position a chair so the reward is just out of reach when you stretch your arm out to the side.

→ When you've finished all the prep, sit in the chair with the right-hand side of your body perpendicular to the countertop. Stretch your right arm towards the treat and keep stretching

WORKS ON ⅂

The shoulders and the muscles of the upper back and sides.

SECRET STASH (EXPLAINED)

Ah, the Secret Stash. It may be potato chips, ice cream, candy or cookies – whatever goodies you have hidden, your heart will skip a happy beat just knowing the stash is safely hidden.

And don't feel bad about your Secret Stash! It's actually crucial to your wellness programme, believe it or not, when used as a reward.

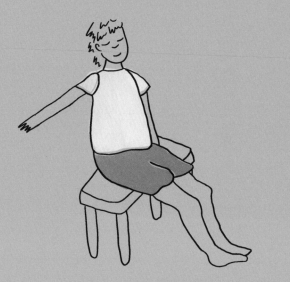

until you can pick it up. Stretch as far as you can before tilting your body. This stretches your middle and lower back muscles and, when you lean, will stretch the muscles on your left-hand side.

→ Once you have your reward, show some self-discipline and put it back, just out of reach again. Big ask.

→ Turn your chair 180 degrees so you are now sitting with your left-hand side to the countertop, and repeat, but this time keep your delicious reward. You've earned it.

#3   The Twist & Bake (or Fake It)

Don't panic – you don't need to bake. You can, though, because you can stretch for the ingredients you need. I've used the fridge in the method below, but cupboards or pantry shelves work just as well.

→ Walk to the fridge with the intention of taking something out of there – maybe milk, yoghurt or a nice cold bottle of wine.

→ Again, preparation is key, so make sure the item you actually want to take from the fridge is accessible, that you know where it is and will actually be able to reach it!

→ Open the fridge door, but instead of facing the contents, you are going to turn away. So, if you want what's inside, then you're going to have to twist!

→ Twist first to the right, turning the whole of your upper body so your head and neck twist as well.

→ Pick up your item, then put it back on the shelf by twisting all the way around and over the left-hand side. Return to facing forwards. This counts as one round of twisting.

→ Start with 5 rounds (then 10 and 20 as you progress). Try to twist every time you go to the fridge or cupboard. It may take effort, but your spine will thank you!

→ FYI, if you have an under-counter fridge, sit on the floor in front and do same spinal twist as above.

Spinal flexibility and the
muscles of the lower back.

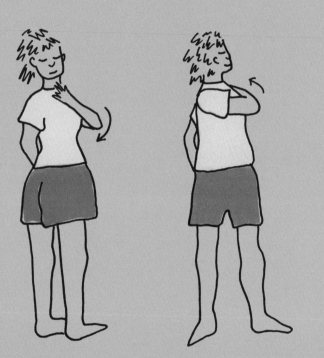

#4 The Nonchalant Stretch

This ingenious stretch will make it look as if you're just hanging out, scrolling through your smartphone or checking your Insta stories, but – just like a graceful swan paddling for all their worth below the surface – what's going on underneath is a whole different story.

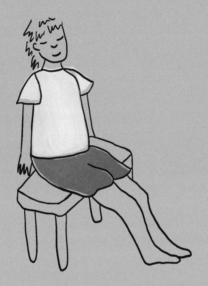

→ Sit nicely at the table with your back and neck straight.

→ Now sit on the edge of the chair with your legs stretched out under the table, heels pressed into the floor and feet pointing upwards.

→ This might require a bit of balance.

→ Allow both arms to just hang by your sides and, when you are ready, flex both your feet upwards from the ankles.

→ Feel that powerful stretch in your calves.

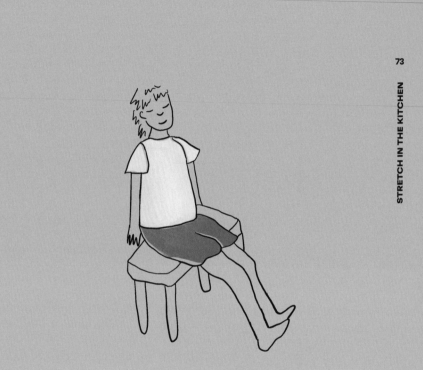

→ Hold for a slow count
of 5 (then 10 and 20
as you progress) before
releasing the hold.

→ Repeat 4 more times –
again, you can increase
this number as you grow
in confidence.

→ This is a great little
stretch that you can
do pretty much anywhere!
You'll look normal from
the waist up, and your
legs will thank you.
Win win.

#5   The Leg Fold Balance

Whether you're an old-school chef or a takeaway lover, there'll always be an element of waiting in the kitchen – a great chance to stretch out your quads, which are those powerful muscles at the top front of both legs.

This stretch can be done almost anywhere and is minimal effort. It's also the stretch you've probably seen serious-looking joggers doing, so you'll look like you mean business too.

Remember, quads can cause problems like knee and back pain if they are overworked or underused, so when it comes to stretching them, it's all about getting the balance right.

→ Stand with both feet planted firmly on the ground, about hip-width apart. It is important you feel stable because this is essentially a balancing stretch.

→ When you are ready, lift your right leg and take hold of the ankle so that you can fold it backwards from the knee.

→ Keeping your balance, keep hold of the ankle and slowly pull your bended right leg up and in towards your right buttock, which will deepen this satisfying stretch.

→ Hold the stretch for a slow count of 5 (then 10 and 20 as you progress).

→ Release your leg and repeat on the other side of the body, bending the left leg at the knee and pulling that bent leg up towards the left buttock.

→ When you have stretched out the quads in both legs, you can rest!

WORKS ON ⌐

The quadriceps.

BALANCING ACT

Good balance helps with posture and co-ordination but might also increase life expectancy – and not just because it reduces the risk of falls.

In a study of people over the age of 50, those who could balance the longest were more likely to be alive a decade later. It also suggested a lower risk of dementia!

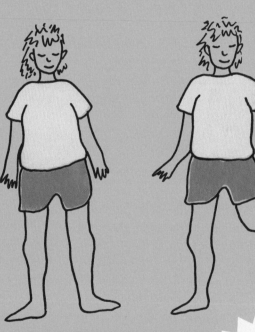

TIP

Once you've mastered standing on one leg, try closing your eyes then standing on tip-toes, which will make your body work harder to stay upright.

Side Leg Swings

This is "double twofer", which just means you work *four* of your target muscle groups with the one flexercise. And what that means is . . . drum roll . . . you get to the end of this series of stretches sooner! Result or what?

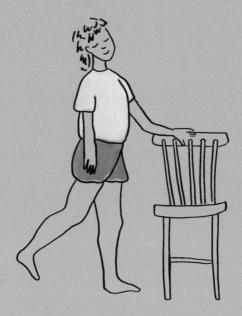

→ Stand up straight alongside a kitchen chair, with your feet hip-width apart.

→ Take a light hold of the back of the chair with your right hand (just to help you stay balanced).

→ Keeping your left leg straight and still, slowly swing your right leg forwards and backwards in one movement.

→ Make the swing as big as you like, and really enjoy the power you can feel from the muscles that are being flexed.

WORKS ON ⏚

The hip flexors and
hamstrings, as well as
the quads and calves.

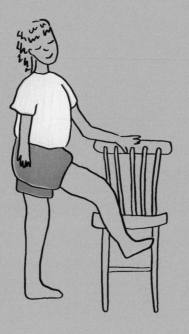

→ Aim to do 10 hip swings
  with the right leg before
  switching sides to do the
  same with the left leg.

→ Notice too how, as you
  build flexibility and
  confidence, you will soon
  be able to increase the
  number of swings you do
  on each side.

→ Your kitchen stretches
  are all done! Go and have
  a well-deserved sit down –
  that washing up can wait.

Stretch at Your Desk

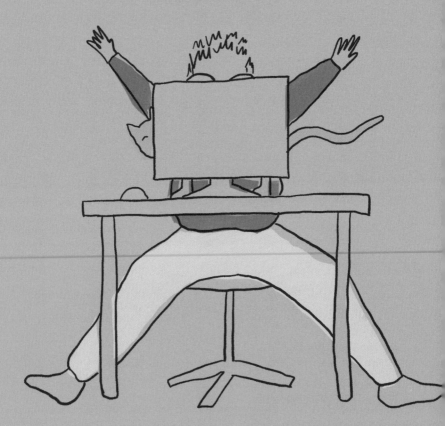

5.

Ah, work. The definition of a necessary evil. Putting aside the long hours, dreaded commute, sadistic bosses and nightmare-inducing office toilets, work is largely responsible for the fact we move our bodies so little and spend so much of our waking time sitting. Well . . . work and Netflix!

The good news for lazy exercisers is that working out at your desk is easy.

If you work at home, you can always step away from your workspace and lie on the floor to stretch out that compressed spine, but if you work in a shared space you may feel a little self-conscious, so all the desk flexercises have been designed to be discreet. At least, more discreet than your colleague's egg sandwich.

#1 Giraffe Stretch

If you've read how much your head weighs (on page 37), you'll understand why, if you only do one desk stretch, you need to channel your inner giraffe and make it this one. Sorry, we're back to inner animals.

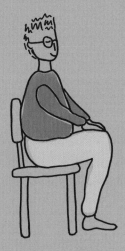

PART 1: STRETCHING THE FRONT OF THE NECK

→ Sit upright in your chair with both feet firmly on the ground. Rest both hands on top of your legs and make sure you are on your sitting bones.

→ Close your eyes and imagine you are a giraffe, with a long neck to reach the treetops. One quick way to get into character is to drop your shoulders down and imagine a thread pulling your head up.

→ You should feel the muscles in your upper back stretching down to help keep your shoulders dropped, which in turn allows the neck to elongate.

→ Stretch your neck, then bring it back to neutral.

→ Hold the stretch for a slow count of 5 (then 10 and 20 as you progress), and release.

WORKS ON ⌐

All the neck muscles.

BALANCING THE BOOKS

There are generations of women who grew up knowing what the word "deportment" meant, and you may have seen images of *nice young ladies* learning to walk properly by balancing a pile of hardback books on their heads. You know what, this is not as bonkers as it sounds!

If you WFH, a great way to stretch your neck between Zoom meetings is to balance a hardback book or two on top of your crown (if you work in the office, it'll still work, but people might think you're weird).

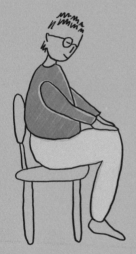

PART 2: STRETCHING THE BACK OF THE NECK

→ Tuck your chin in towards the body and allow the back of the neck to lengthen. It's important to keep the neck strong and straight as possible.

→ Once you have this perfect alignment, hold the stretch for a slow count of 5 (then 10 and 20 as you progress). Release.

Shrug It Off

If it helps you get into character for this one, imagine someone coming at you with penetrating (and pointless) questions about the universe or the meaning of life and, in your mind's eye, see yourself just shrugging your reply. Now do it for real.

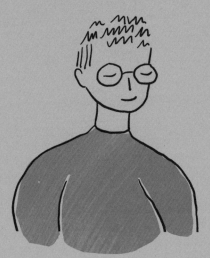

→ Sit upright in your work chair, with your spine straight and your feet flat on the ground.

→ Rest both hands on the tops of your legs, palms facing down, and close your eyes.

→ Now, lift both shoulders up towards your ears, raising them as high as you can.

→ Once both shoulders are at the full extent of that stretch just drop them both back down.

WORKS ON ↴

The shoulders and their supporting muscles.

THE POWER OF MANTRA

Here's a short mantra to help you through this simple shoulder stretch. Repeat after me: "Don't ask me!" Or, if you are super busy (you are at work, after all) and pressed for time, try "Huh?", which works just as well!

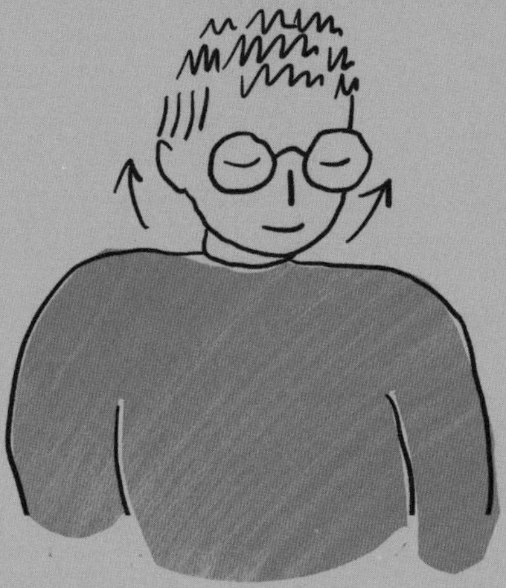

→ Exaggerate the drop and as soon as you've done that, raise both shoulders again.

→ It helps if you co-ordinate your breathing with this flexercise, so inhale as you lift both shoulders and exhale loudly as you drop them again. Repeat 10 times (then 20 and 50 as you progress).

#3 Easy Chair Bends

The advantage of this stretch is that you can pretend you're picking up a dropped pencil if anyone catches you.

Quick tip first: if you want to avoid concussion, you'll need to move your chair sideways on to your desk, which will give you the space to fold forwards.

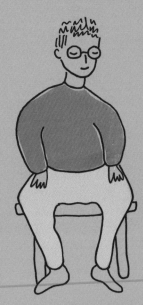

→ When you are ready to stretch, move your body so that you are perching on the edge of your work chair with your knees bent, legs wide apart and both feet flat on the floor.

→ Keeping your knees bent, breathe in and as you exhale bring the upper part of your body down to meet your thighs. If you can, rest your palms on the floor between your legs.

WORKS ON ↴

The whole of the back and the muscles of the inner thighs.

AFTER-LUNCH TIP

Folding the body in half squeezes all the internal organs of the digestive tract, so if you are in the office and you've been out for a hearty lunch, you may want to skip this flexercise and do it in the morning!

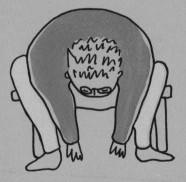

→ With your body folded in half, rest in this position for a slow count of 5 (then 10 and 20 as you progress).

→ When you are done, inhale and slowly unfold yourself. Repeat this folding flexercise 5 times (then 10 and 20 as you progress).

→ And rest . . . or do some actual work!

Nose-to-Knee Stretch

If you wear lace-up shoes for this one, if anyone passes your desk when you are mid flow with this flexercise, you can make like you're just tying your laces.

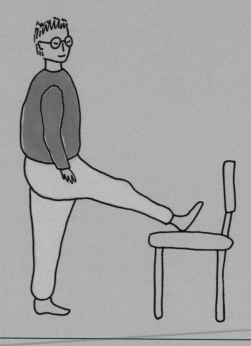

→ Begin by swivelling your work chair around so the back is away from you, then stand in front of it with your legs shoulder-width apart.

→ With your knees soft and slightly bent, lift your upper body and tilt your pelvis slightly forward.

→ Keep your shoulders down and raise your right leg to rest it on the chair.

→ Place both hands on your right thigh, just above the kneecap, and keep your left leg straight.

→ Slowly inhale and begin to lower your upper body towards your right thigh.

WORKS ON ⅂

The whole of the backs of the
legs, stretching the hamstrings
and the calves making it
another "twofer" flexercise.

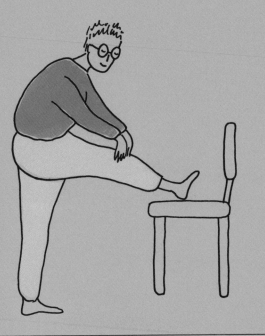

→   Allow the body to fold
    forwards, and you should
    feel the stretch in those
    muscles at the back of
    your leg.

→   Stay down in the folded
    position for a slow count
    of 5 (then 10 and 20 as
    you progress). Breathe
    slowly and deeply in this

position, allowing
the body to relax into
a deeper fold with each
out breath.

→   When you are done, lift
    your upper body, take
    your right leg off the
    chair and repeat the
    exact same flexercise
    on the left-hand side.

#5   Sock Stock Check

You can just breath normally through this flexercise, which is all about encouraging the hips to open out.

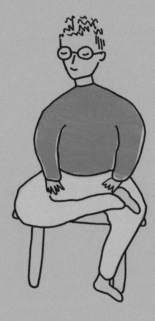

→ Sit upright in your work chair with your legs apart, feet planted on the floor.

→ Now lift your right leg to bring your right ankle up to rest on your left knee.

→ Cradle your right ankle and right foot in both hands and really feel the stretch in the right hip.

→ Hold this stretch for 2 minutes (or longer if you are able). If you get bored, do a sock stock check. Are you still wearing both socks? Do they match? Are they clean? Are they even yours? You'll be surprised how quickly the time flies . . .

WORKS ON ↴

Loosening tight hips, so you'll be "The One" (there's always One) sitting in lotus position at your next yoga class.

PROBLEMS CAUSED BY TOO TIGHT HIPS

— You'll never be "The One" sitting in full lotus in your yoga class
— Leg cramps and sore muscles, especially in the upper legs

— Unexplained knee pains
— Early signs of spine curvature
— Lower back pain and neck pain

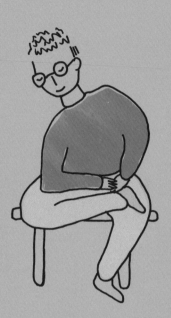

→ When you feel ready, you can deepen this stretch by bending your right arm so that you can rest your elbow on your right knee. Apply a gentle pressure through the elbow to push the knee down. Feel how that deepens the stretch? You should now be able to feel the stretch moving deep into the buttocks.

→ As you grow in confidence, you can extend it even further by bending the upper body forwards as you use the elbow to push the right knee down.

→ After several minutes stretching out the right hip, switch over and repeat the exact same stretches to the left hip.

#6 The "I Think Better Standing" Stretch

You're deep in thought, solving a crisis or coming up with your company's genius next move. At least, that's what everyone will think as you stand there, looking wise and powerful.

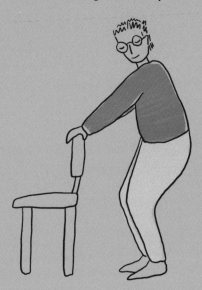

→ Stand behind your chair, making sure you are close enough to hold onto the top of the backrest. This is your prop.

→ Your feet should be flat on the ground and shoulder-width apart.

→ Bend your knees slightly and take hold of the back of the chair with both hands. Slowly bend your upper body forwards until your back is parallel to the floor. Your arms should now be at a 90-degree angle to your legs.

→ Lower your body towards the floor while still holding on the back of the chair. Feel just how deeply that stretches the muscles in both legs.

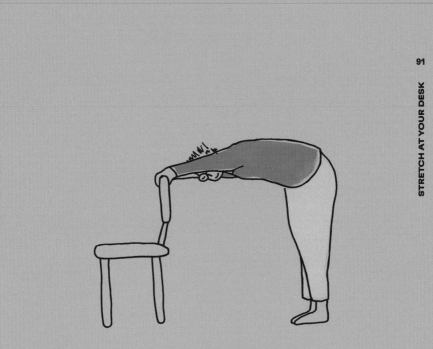

→ When you have lowered the body as far as it can go, rest and breathe slowly and deeply.

→ Hold this position for a slow count of 5 (then 10 and 20 as you progress) before standing.

→ If your chair is on wheels then tuck it under the desk so it doesn't roll away when you lean on it.

→ That's it for the desk stretches! Your colleagues will marvel at your new-found flexibility (probably).

Stretch on the Move

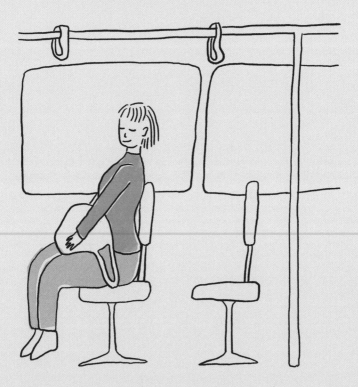

6.

These simple flexercises work whenever you are on the move – travelling by car, bus, train or plane. But be warned: you might cause an international incident if you try them while riding a desert camel.

Space is usually restricted when we are on the move – and then there's the added risk of scaring your fellow passengers or drivers if you start throwing your weight around at the traffic lights – so discretion here has also been built in for your protection. Your stretching secret is safe with me.

#1 Eye Palming

If you are not driving or in charge of any moving form of transportation, then try this soothing exercise on any long journey. (If you are driving, wait until you're parked up somewhere safe, obviously.)

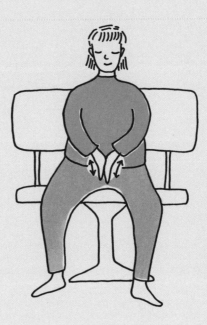

→ Rub the palms of your hands together until you can feel some heat generating between them. You may need to rub vigorously!

→ Close your eyes and gently rest the right palm over the right eye and the left palm over the left eye.

→ Feel the heat and warmth being transmitted to the eye muscles, which will begin to relax.

WORKS ON ↲

Tired eyes and will help
relieve tension headaches.

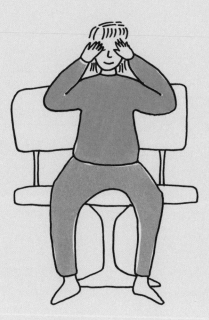

→ When you feel all the
heat and energy has
drained away, keep your
eyes closed and lower
your hands so you can
rub your palms together
again to create more
heat and energy.

→ Repeat this 5 times, and
increase the number of
repetitions if you are
stuck in a bad traffic jam
or on the runway waiting
for take-off.

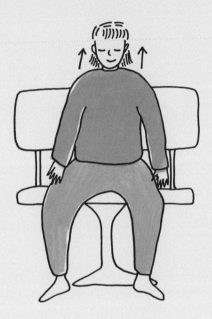

→ Try and sit as upright
   as you can in your car/
   plane/train/bus/tram/
   ferry seat.

→ Keep your arms hanging
   loosely alongside
   the body.

→ Inhale and lift both
   your shoulders up towards
   your ears - really
   use the muscles of the
   upper back to get both
   shoulders up as high
   as you can.

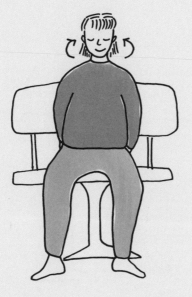

→ Now, keeping them raised, slowly roll both shoulders back, squeezing the shoulder blades tightly together.

→ Exhale and drop both shoulders back to their normal resting position.

→ Repeat the backwards shoulder roll 5 times, then do the same lift and drop 5 more times but rolling both shoulders forwards.

3

Rising Trot in Your Seat

If you're on horseback then the horse is doing the "rising" bit for you, but your lower back will still be getting a great workout!

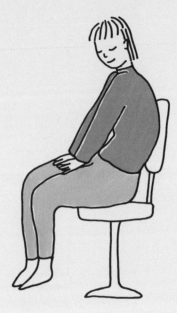

→ Sit upright in your seat and rest both hands on the tops of your thighs, palms down.

→ Now, inhale and flex your spine forwards by pushing your chest out and up. You will feel this in the middle and lower portions of your back.

→ This is a dynamic flex, so we're not hanging around between movements.

WORKS ON ⤵

Lower back, but flexes
the whole spine.

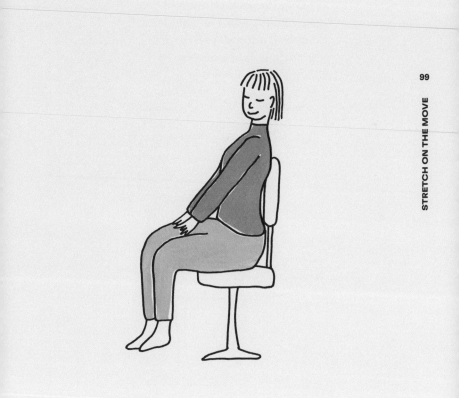

→ As you exhale, snap the
torso and upper chest
back to the starting
position and keep this
back and forth movement
going. If you know
anything about horse
riding, this flexercise
will feel like the rising
trot it is named after.

→ Keep your eyes closed
to help you stay focused
on the spine.

→ You can do this easy
flexercise for 1 minute
or 5 - it's up to you.

4

Toes Meet Ankle

If you've worked your way through the stretches in Chapter Five (Stretch at Your Desk), then you already know all about the power of a simple foot flex, and you can make this one as discreet (or not) as space allows.

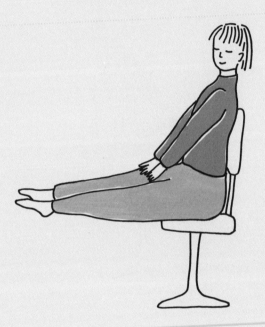

→ If you can, stretch both legs out in front of you to create a 90-degree angle with the floor. You'll soon feel a big stretch on the calves and hamstrings too.

→ Now, flex both feet back in towards the body.

→ You should be flexing at the ankles, so this stretch is good for those often-overlooked but important joints too.

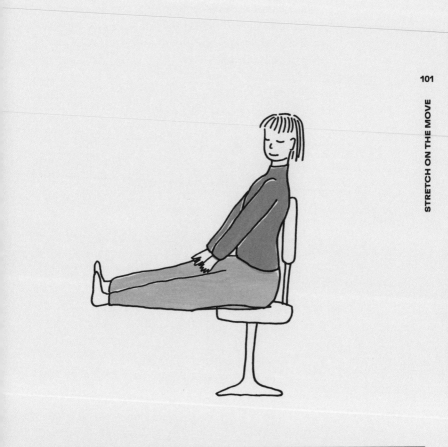

→ If you are travelling in a confined space – or shy about drawing the attention of fellow travellers – keep your heels on the ground and flex the feet from that position. You'll still get a good stretch of the calves, but less of one for the hamstrings.

5

The "Hover Leg" Stretch

Your fellow travellers won't look twice at someone who's simply crossing their legs. If they did look closer, though, they'd probably mistake you for some kind of Jedi, as you're actually *hovering* one leg over the other.

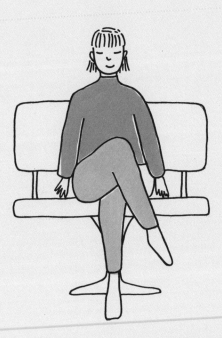

→ Sit with your spine straight and your arms hanging loosely by your sides.

→ Lift your right leg and bring it over your left leg as if you were about to rest it there. Instead, keep your right leg lifted and let it hover above your left leg.

WORKS ON ⤵

The hamstrings.

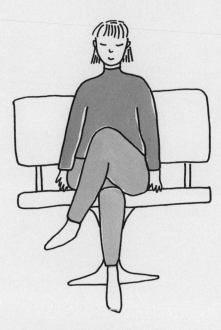

→ You will quickly feel a strong stretch in the hamstring muscle at the back of your right leg and may struggle to keep the leg raised for more than a few seconds.

→ Build up to a hold of a slow count of 5 (then 10 and 20 as you progress).

→ Repeat the Hover Leg Stretch by raising your left leg and keeping it hovering above the right.

6

Give Your Knees Some Love

You will need space in front of you to raise your knee and hug it, so you might need to push the car seat back to get that extra space. If you're on public transport, you should be fine.

Remember the golden rule of symmetry: if you stretch out one side of the body, you need to stretch out the other in the same way and for the same amount of time

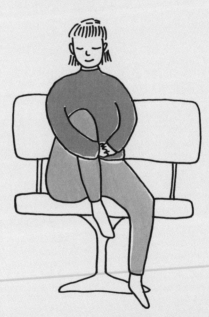

→ Lift your right knee up and clasp both hands around it so you can hug it into your chest.

→ Hold and count slowly to 5 (then 10 and 20 as you progress).

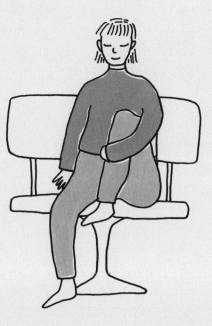

→ Repeat with the
   other leg. Couldn't
   be simpler.

On-the-Edge Stretch

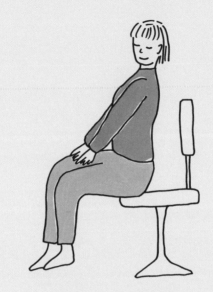

→ Shimmy to the edge of your seat and lift both feet so you are on your tiptoes (or you would be, if you were standing).

→ Bend your knees and, at the same time, tuck the raised feet in behind you, as far as the space and your balance will allow!

→ Now imagine you are about to start dropping to your knees. As you lower them, feel the stretch to the quadriceps muscles that run from your thigh to your knee at the front of your leg.

→ You are lowering your knees, but you are not bringing them to the ground. Try to find the sweet spot between slipping off the edge of the seat and using the muscles of the legs and abdomen to keep you balanced.

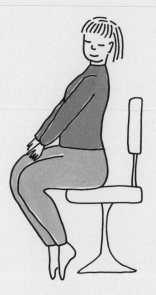

→ Once you've found it,
count slowly to 5 (then 10
and 20 as you progress),
then come back to sitting
fully in your seat.

→ This manoeuvre makes
the lower spine work
hard too, so when you
are finished, go back
to Exercise 3 in this
chapter (see page 98) to
counter that by releasing
any tension that has
built up around the
lower back.

→ With that, our on-the-
move stretching journey
is over, which means
we're getting near the
end. Trust me, I'm as sad
as you are. So without
further ado . . .

Stretch While Doing Other Things

(like brushing your teeth
or waiting for the kettle to boil)

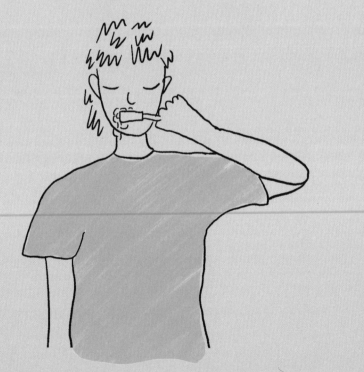

7.

One of the best ways to integrate movement and regular stretching into our daily lives is to do it when you're busy doing something else.

Some folk call this "multitasking" and pretend it's a special gift from the gods that they've been born with.

It's not, and they weren't. With a bit of practice, anyone can do it – even the laziest exerciser!

#1   Cleaning Your Teeth

Works on the lower back, neck and shoulders.

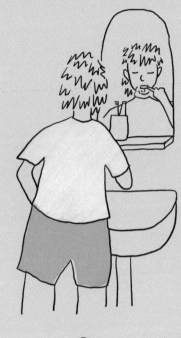

❶

The Twist and Bake (or Fake It)

Exercise 3,
In the Kitchen

(page 70)

❷

Head Grab

Exercise 1,
In the Kitchen

(page 66)

❸

The Circle Stretch

Exercise 2,
On the Move

(page 96)

VARIATION — face away from the mirror to do these, and twist around to spit.

#2 Ironing

Works on the neck, shoulders, core and quadriceps.

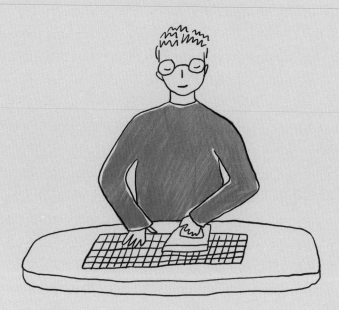

1

Starfish and Swan

Exercise 2, In Bed

(page 16)

SAFETY NOTE — keep your eyes on the hot iron and its position at all times!

2

Reach and Reward

Exercise 2, In the Kitchen

(page 68)

VARIATION — Put your tea or coffee (or, let's be honest, wine) safely on a heat-resistant surface nearby (and almost out of reach) so you have to work to get to it every time you want to take a sip!

3

The "I Think Better Standing" Stretch

Exercise 6, At Your Desk

(page 91)

#3 Waiting For a Saucepan /Kettle to Boil

Works the legs, hips and back.

STRETCH WHILE DOING OTHER THINGS

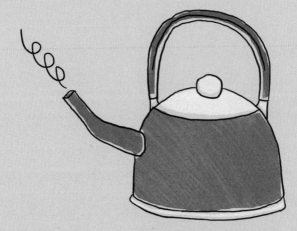

 ❶
Side Leg Swings

Exercise 6,
In the Kitchen

(page 76)

❷
Give Your Knees Some Love

Exercise 6,
On the Move

(page 104)

 ❸
Easy Chair Bends

Exercise 3,
At Your Desk

(page 84)

You'll need to be standing sideways on to the countertop.

Try to increase the pace of these as you get into a rhythm.

#4 Putting the Grocery Shopping Away

Works the back, inner thighs and neck.

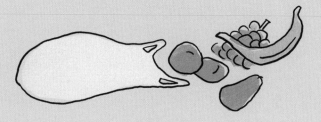

1

Easy Chair Bends

Exercise 3,
At Your Desk

(page 84)

VARIATION — simply adapt this stretch so you're standing instead!

2

Giraffe Stretch

Exercise 1,
At Your Desk

(page 80)

VARIATION — As you'll be standing (not sitting) and raising your arms, this will lengthen your neck and the muscles in your upper back as you reach up to put the groceries away in the cupboard. Reach for the highest shelves!

3

The Twist and Bake (or Fake It)

Exercise 3,
In the Kitchen

(page 70)

Good for fridge goods and those higher shelves where you'll need to twist and reach up to store your shopping.

Hanging the Washing Out to Dry

Works the legs, back and quadriceps.

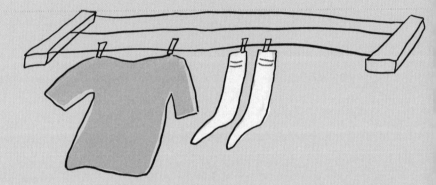

❶ Easy Chair Bends

Exercise 3,
At Your Desk

(page 84)

VARIATION — simply adapt this stretch so you're standing instead!

❷ Side Leg Swings

Exercise 6,
In the Kitchen

(page 76)

You can always wear dark glasses and a big hat if you're worried about what the neighbours might think.

❸ The Leg Fold Balance

Exercise 5,
In the Kitchen

(page 74)

Perch on one leg while hanging up the washing, using one hand to hold your other leg – like a magnificent flamingo.

Putting the Bins Out

Works the upper back.

❶

Rotating Chicken Wings

Exercise 1,
In the Bath

(page 32)

Give the neighbours something
to talk about and strut back to your
front door rotating your shoulders
like a happy chicken!

Stretch Your Breath and Exercise Your Mind

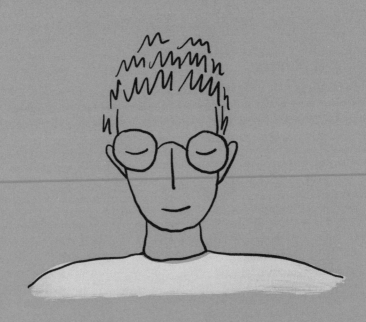

8.

MEET YOUR BREATH

Set a timer now for just one minute.
Sit quietly away from any distractions.
Close your eyes and count how many
times you breath in and out during that
one minute.

How many times did you breathe
without consciously trying to change
the pattern of your breath?

15–20 times?
10–15 times?
6–8 times?

The "normal" respiration rate for an
adult at rest is 12–20 times, but there are
many benefits of slowing the breath more
than that.

As well as lowering your heart rate and
blood pressure, longer, slower and deeper
breathing can also help tackle
or improve anxiety, stress, concentration
and focus, recovery rate from exercise and
fractured sleep patterns.

If you are new to thinking about your
breath, this simple exercise will help connect
you to the way you breath naturally. That
said, as soon as we start to think about
breathing our breath will automatically slow
down and deepen. That's already half way
to stretching it, so this couldn't be easier
or more rewarding to do!

1

Hand Tracing Breath Exercise

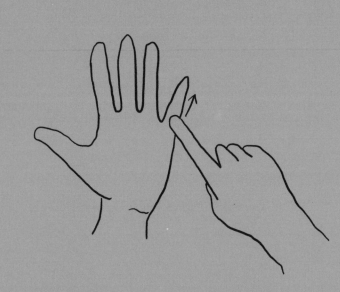

→ Place the index finger of one hand on the outside of the "pinkie" finger on your other hand. As you breathe in, trace up to the tip of your "pinkie", and as you breathe out, trace down the inside of your "pinkie".

→ On your next inhale, trace up the inside of your ring finger, and on the exhale, trace down the outside of your ring finger.

When you've finished this exercise, repeat the Breath Counting exercise we started this chapter with. Now see how many times you breath in one minute. Has it changed?

→ Inhale and trace up the outside of your middle finger; exhale and trace down the inside of your middle finger.

→ Continue finger by finger until you've traced your entire hand.

→ Now, reverse the whole process and trace from your thumb back to your "pinkie" finger keeping your breath steady and the tracing pattern in a nice, even flow.

2

Box Your Breath

Once we've connected with the breath, we can learn to control it ready to stretch it. Again, find a quiet place to sit and make sure you won't be disturbed or distracted.

Close your eyes and follow the steps below to "box" your breath and also learn how to "suspend" it.

→ With your eyes closed, breath in, to a slow and silent count of 4.

→ Keeping your eyes closed, hold your breath for a slow count of 4.

→ Exhale and release your breath for the same slow count of 4.

→ At the end of the exhale, suspend your breath for a slow count of 4.

AFTERWARDS ⬎

When you've finished this exercise, again repeat the Breath Counting exercise (see page 117) we started this chapter with and now see how many times you breath in one minute.

PAYING ATTENTION TO THE BREATH

How do you feel as your breathing slows down?

Does your inhale easily match your exhale, or do you find it easier to breath out than to breath in?

If you are struggling to connect more deeply to your breath put your hands on your tummy and notice how, as you breath in, your stomach pushes out into your hands and how as you breath in, your tummy contracts again.

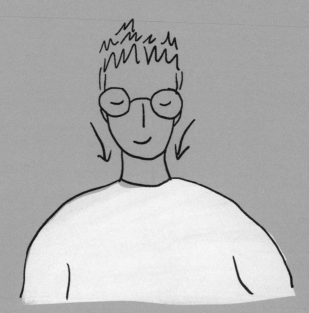

→ With practice, you will find your breath settles happily into this rhythm and you can then begin to experiment with stretching the breath itself by increasing the count from four to 5 and eventually all the way up to 10 or even beyond.

#3 Stretch Your Breath

Practice slowing, deepening and stretching your breath whenever you can.

You can do this sitting in the car or on the train, in the bath or in bed before you fall asleep and you'll quickly discover that the more you pay attention to your pattern of breathing, the easier you will find it to slow and stretch the breath at will.

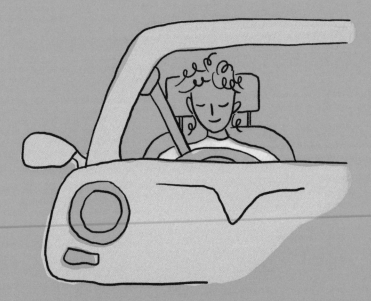

EXERCISING YOUR 'THINKING CAP' (AKA THE MIND)

This doesn't just mean doing Wordle every day, although that won't hurt! Scientists at Harvard University have reported that people who meditate daily for 40 minutes a day have bigger brains than those who don't.

The researchers were astonished to discover that people who meditate have increased thickness in those parts of the brain that deal with attention and processing sensory information, and also of those areas that are important for our emotional processing (thinking) and wellness.

This flies in the face of biology and the normal aging process which would see these areas – including the part of the brain known as our Thinking Cap – grow thinner not thicker with age!

And here's what's really great about this discovery: if you can sit still for a while and breathe, then you too can meditate.

#4   How To Meditate
and Stretch Your Mind

**Believe it or not, you can do this
in just 6 easy steps.**

→ Find somewhere quiet to
sit. Set a timer on your
smartphone for just 5
minutes (you can build up
to a longer meditation).

→ Find a comfortable seated
position, then notice
how your body is today.

→ Focus on your breath.
Use any of the exercises
in this chapter to help
you connect to your
breathing.

→ Notice how quickly and how
much your mind wanders.
The mind hates stillness
and will do anything it
can to get you up and back
into your busy life. So,
thank it for helping you
to cope with everyday life
but ask it to step down
for a while.

→ Practise kindness towards
yourself and don't get
frustrated with your
wandering mind. It thinks
it is helping, which it
normally would be! Just
keep bringing yourself
back to your focus on
the breath.

→ And that's it! When the
timer goes off, thank
yourself for exercising
your mind.

→ You've done your first
meditation, and you
can build up to the
40 minutes a day that
research shows helps
the brain and the mind
to grow!

When you've finished this exercise,
again repeat the Breath Counting
exercise we started this chapter
with and now see how many times
you breath in 1 minute.

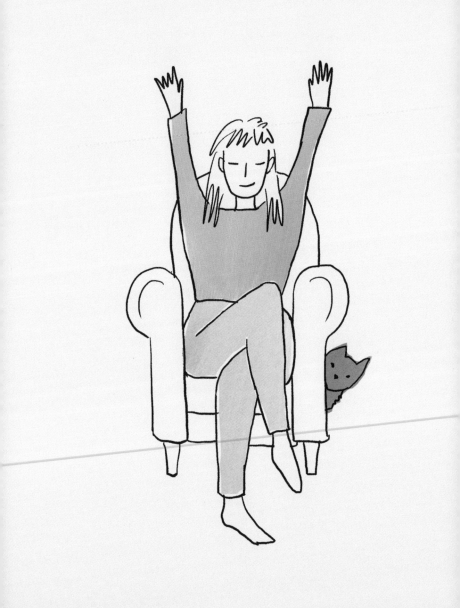

ABOUT THE AUTHOR

Susan is a wellness and self-help writer who specialises in shining a light on those topics that can help people overcome their physical, mental and spiritual challenges to live their best lives. She has studied esoteric traditions in India and the UK. Susan lives in Yorkshire.

ACKNOWLEDGEMENTS

With thanks to my publisher, Kate Pollard, for her vision of a book that could help us all get out of our heads and moving a little more, without even having to leave the comfort of our homes. Genius! Thanks also to my editor, Matt Tomlinson, for bringing a gentle humour to the proceedings. If you're breathing then, in my book, you're already doing great — better than great, in fact — so thanks to all those who have stopped to share a breath or two with me along the winding way. They already know who they are, and why they matter to me.

Published in 2022 by OH Editions
Part of Welbeck Publishing Group.
Based in London and Sydney.
www.welbeckpublishing.com

Design © 2022 OH Editions

Text © 2022 Susan Elizabeth Clark
Illustrations © 2022 Evi-O.Studio

A CIP catalogue record for this
book is available from the British
Library.

ISBN 978-1-91431-792-7

Publisher: Kate Pollard
Editor: Matt Tomlinson
Art Direction & Design: Evi-O.
Studio | Susan Le
Design Assistant & Illustration |
Katherine Zhang
Production: Arlene Alexander

Printed and bound by RR Donnelley
in China.

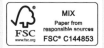

MIX
Paper from
responsible sources
FSC® C144853

10 9 8 7 6 5 4 3 2 1

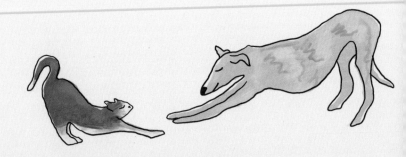